WORDS TO LIVE BY
Whatever you're up against, this book's for you.
by Ann Murray Paige

www.annmurraypaige.com
Copyright 2011. All rights reserved.

Also by Ann Murray Paige and available at
www.annmurraypaige.com:

-pink tips. breast cancer advice from someone who's been there.
-More Words To Live By.
-Words To Live By: The Early Years.
-The Face Of Breast-less America. A Memoir (Summer, 2012)
-<u>The Breast Cancer Diaries</u> DVD

AUTHOR'S NOTE
May 12, 2011 10:32 AM

I have compiled these blogs for two reasons: the first, in response to those who want "to read my book." I ask, "what book?" and they answer, "the book of your blogs." The second is my mother, who at 84 years old has no computer and no desire to get one, but desperately wants to read her daughter's blog.

The purpose of writing for me is to release--the tension, the fear and the funniness of life with two children, a husband, a dog, and metastatic breast cancer. When I was originally diagnosed with breast cancer at age 38 in 2004, I did all I could to beat back the beast--prophylactic bilateral mastectomy without reconstruction-- (yes, that's not a typo, it does read with*out*) dose-dense chemotherapy (the double shots) and 25 rounds of radiation. I lived 6 years until a strange sound in my left lung confirmed that the breast cancer was back and had traveled into my lung--now called "metastatic". Not that I wasn't inspired before to write but with my future literally hanging in the balance of medicines, body scans and lunch boxes I have dug deep into what it really means *to live.*

Words To Live By is the first in a series of blog anthologies from my writing at ProjectPinkDiary.com. These entries, from September, 2010--days before my surprise re-diagnosis of breast cancer, through the spring of 2011--are meant to inspire, educate and in some cases instill a laugh. Take them to the beach, to the waiting room, on the plane or in the hammock. I'm glad to share this time with you.

And I wish you the very best of health. *-Ann Murray Paige*

FOR MY MOTHER, MARY JANE.
NOW YOU CAN READ MY BLOGS, MOM.

TABLE OF CONTENTS
September, 2010-April, 2011

PINK RIBBONS AND WHY THEY MATTER
September 30, 2010 12:22:14 PM

On the eve of Breast Cancer Awareness Month, I wanted to make a strong shout out to all the people reading this blog who care about breast cancer.

I think it could be quite easy to see the pink ribbons donning soup cans from Montana to Mississippi, California to the Carolinas, to the cute little Mom n' Pop stores that dot the beautiful Maine landscape and get a bit sick of them. I know they're everywhere--what do they really mean?

I'm here to put a face to those pink ribbons: they mean me.

And they mean my friend Raychel whose mother and sister both died of the disease. And my pal Brooke's mother who fought and won her battle and is sitting somewhere in Ohio making a sandwich and thanking her lucky stars she made it through. Those ribbons are a woman named Michele whom I've never met, but who like thousands of others who've been affected by breast cancer and who support my non-profit Project Pink or have seen my film *"The Breast Cancer Diaries"* and can relate to everything I'm living through and write to me at my website. It's all of us--and so many more--the 1 in every 8 women who are diagnosed with breast cancer each year in the United States.

I know it seems like "the Pink" is everywhere in October, but so are we. We are walking down your street, driving the car you just passed, smiling at you from a toll booth, standing next to you at the grocery store as you pick up that soup can.

And we, all of us, thank you for any and every thing you do--from cancer walks to non-profit donations to buying that ridiculous soup can-- to donate to the cause of making breast cancer go away.

Believe me, nobody more than me would like to see that silly pink can of soup--and the reason for it--disappear forever.

MY CANCER IS BACK
October 21, 2010 03:14:01 PM

It's been a while since I blogged and for those of you who are wondering if everything's okay, well--no. About a week ago I got the surprising and personally earth-shattering news that my cancer has come back.

I want to say that finding my breast cancer has returned during Breast Cancer Awareness Month is taking the theme a little too far, and I hadn't intended to do so--not this month, not last October, nor any of the 6 October's I've lived, calling myself a "survivor" since my original diagnosis back in 2004. I really thought I'd beaten it.

But like all cancer "survivors", the survivor is a misnomer. It's more like a hope, a prayer, a wish, a cry, it's what we all believe we are, because we must live in faith and optimism. Yet the reality is that if you've had cancer it can always come back--anytime, any place---and if you're like me, knock you on your backside with sadness, discouragement and sheer terror.

I truly thought the double mastectomy-no-reconstruction-dose-dense-chemo-radiation-tamoxifen cocktail I sipped all summer long back in '04 would have beaten back the beast. But here I go again, talking to doctors, writing down notes, hugging my kids, collapsing on my husband, and trying like hell to save my life--AGAIN.

So to all of you who pray, pray.
To all of you who chant, chant.
To all of you who vibe with the universe, vibe.
And if you're like some people I know who find God in different places, I ask that you send out a holler in my name to that God.

I knew someone who used to sit in a duck blind on a chilly Maine morning with his steaming cup of coffee, looking around at the beautiful earth and golden sunrise and feel God. I am asking him and all the rest of you who have faith in anything, anything, to have some faith for me too.

I am a fighter and I plan to win--with good medications, great doctors, amazing friends, a strong family,

and Faith--from any and everywhere I can get it.

PUTTING THE 'ER' IN CANCER
Nov 5, 2010 03:38 PM

It's been a month to the day that my doctor told me the breast cancer I beat back 6 years ago has returned. This is a lousy anniversary to celebrate. But celebrate something I must, because sitting around letting recurrent breast cancer make me insane with worry and fear is not my idea of living.

It's hard not to be scared, though, when you hit the Emergency Room of the local hospital 4 times in 8 days–which I did last month–twice for BC complications and twice for the-massage-that-was-supposed-to-relax-me-just-put-my-shoulder-into-spasm reasons. And for fun and breathing, I had to go again last night when the sore throat I had at 3 p.m. turned into a full blown flu at 10 p.m. and rendered my lungs almost useless. Not a good sleeping plan.

By now I know the people at the ER by site and some by name. As soon as I pull into the driveway and park the car they're practically waving me in. I know the intake nurse, the front desk personnel and at least three of the doctors by "She's ba-a-a-ack.'" The name of the poor fellow who blew my IV line 3 times I'll try to forget–but it's quite something when you know enough to tell him use the baby butterfly with the 3CC syringe or else the blood will hemolyze. A month ago I couldn't spell hemolyze much less define it. This is when you know you've come to the ER a wee bit too often.

I promise you though that despite the sticks and blown lines, the needles into my shoulder, the MRI's, CT scans and the countess X-Rays, I am still here. I am still kicking, I am still fighting—and I plan to kick cancer's BUTT. It's that simple.

I will get to a point where I am out there having fun again, living my precious, good life. And then the people at the ER can wave to me as I drive past their entrance on my way to enjoying a new anniversary—the one that will celebrate how many months (years!) it's been since I've had to go to the ER.

Now there's a milestone worth celebrating.

HOLDING MY BREATH
Nov 15, 2010 12:46 PM

A good friend wanted to know, "how did you find out the cancer came back?"

I find myself holding my breath as I write this. I haven't talked about that until now. Some days, I hate allowing the cancer any space at all. Some mornings I wake up and pretend for as long as I can that I don't even have it. Other days I figure if I don't talk about the C, it will have less oxygen to survive inside of me. Or maybe it's the more verbal oxygen I give it, the more it lives on? Either way, these wandering thoughts are a look-see into the spinning mind of a recurrent BC woman–me- and today I decided to get past the superstition and jump on this cancer's back and spit it out. Spit out all that it's trying to do so that in exposing it, I knock it down and out.

So here's how it went: my oncologist, on a routine visit, felt that she couldn't hear as much air whooshing through my left lung as she could my right. Since my left breast is where the breast cancer started, she got worried–and sent me for an x-ray. The x-ray showed a thickening in that lung area, so she sent me for a pet scan. The pet scan revealed the cancer. Weeks later a test confirmed that it was not a new cancer, but the old cancer come back.

At the same time I had some pain in my back, I wasn't really able to lie down flat to sleep and I was scheduled for an MRI to find out if my hereditary back issues were flaring up. After the pet scan showed what it showed, I realized that my back was reacting to what was happening in my lungs.

So there it is: the beginning of this next part of my life. After a few weeks of mind-numbing fear and confusion over which pills to try first (and a few trips to the ER) I am on Tamoxifen again plus ovarian suppression. We'll see if it's working–and here's the tricky part–in 6 to 9 more weeks. Yup, I have to wait that long. It takes that long for the medicine to show that it's working–3 months in total. That's a lot of breath holding.

So if you see me walking down the street purposely not talking about cancer, you'll know why. I'm either starving it of oxygen or else I'm pretending it's not me who's up against this beast again. Either way, give me a smile or a hug and know that whatever happens I'll keep writing.

There's no lost oxygen in that–except what I'm breathing in for me.

I WILL IF I HAVE TO
Nov 18, 2010 11:39 PM

The trick about this new cancer I face is that I don't know what else to do to stop it.

I did everything, I mean EVERYTHING, to get rid of it the first time: bilateral mastectomy with no reconstruction, dose dense (double strength) chemotherapy, radiation and tamoxifen for the recommended 5 years. Other than walk through a radioactive nuclear plant in my bathing suit or drink chemo from a juice box, I'm not sure I could have done any other medical thing to help myself.

I always ate right–organic when I could, lots of fruits and veggies, limited alcohol and attempts at cutting down on sweets. But like the average Joe, I also partake of the nectar of life. I sneak cookies that my sister Joan bakes (which should be in bakeries across the country they're so good), I enjoy a good bottle of JR Cohen cab when invited by friends, and I LOVE my Dunkies coffee. Does this make me unhealthy? I never thought so–and clearly, none of the other regular folks out there who enjoy these treats of life alongside me are facing recurrent breast cancer.

So what's the deal with me?

I don't know–but clearly I need to find out. Time is of the essence. Who knows how much I have left? I'll tell you one thing: I'll be damned if I'm going to find out.

Do I want to give up the fun things in my life? Before when I had breast cancer, the answer was no. In fact, hell no–because what else did I learn from my scare but that life was too short–so enjoy it while I can?

But now, it's different. Now I am running for my life. And I am not running away as much as I am rushing toward something–anything that may save me.

I read books, I scan the internet, I take advice from people, but to be honest, it's overwhelming. Avocados–good! Avocados–bad. Coconut oil–good! Coconut oil–bad. Dairy–bad? Soy? We're not sure yet. I'm going crazy deciphering what may help me, Ann Murray Paige, starve off this breast cancer in my body and make it go away for good.

But I'm on the hunt. I will figure it out. But yes it drives me nuts (Nuts–good!) to feel so lost in the grocery store of my life. To offset that, I search for the bright side. Like–I don't have to have another bilateral mastectomy—good! I don't have to have chemotherapy immediately (there are hormone therapies that work for breast cancer)–good!

And let's not forget the best bright side of them all– I didn't have to walk through a nuclear plant in my bathing suit–good!

But I will if I have to.

THE SURVIVOR MISNOMER AND WHY WE NEED IT

Nov 23, 2010 08:18 PM

A week or two after I heard that the breast cancer I fought off 6 years ago was back, I found myself meandering through the girls section of Marshall's trying to forget about my life for awhile. As I felt the velvet and ruffles of a cute little jumper my text bell went off. I looked down and it was a dear friend of mine from the mid-coast area.

"Any news?"

She was waiting to hear–as I had been–whether this was my original breast cancer returned or a new cancer that had developed.

"It's my original BC."

Her next text came from a confused place, a place I'd been as well.

"So the same cancer can come back to a new location after you beat it? I'm sorry it's hard for me to understand."

My response began with "join the club."

Before I got this recurrence, I never liked the term "survivor" of cancer for this very reason. It's a misnomer to say you've survived cancer because the reality is you

don't ever beat it. You get it under control. Cancer is a
devil–it can hide out in tiny molecules that the best of
diagnostic tools can't detect. The docs can get what they
think is all of it, and tell you that, but really–you know
you've beaten it when you die of something else. How's
that for a prognosis?

Yet as I looked at this text I actually realized something:
we cancer people have to believe we are survivors. I mean,
if you're not a survivor what are you? You're a victim.
You're a target. Or you're dead.

And we are not dead.

We are still here, we are alive, we are working, walking,
loving, living– we breast cancer, prostate cancer, lung
cancer ETC. "recipients" as I've been known to call us, we
ARE. And we are fighting off this hidden beast with
everything we've got.

If that isn't the definition of survivor, I don't know what is.

CANCEL MY CASKET
Nov 29, 2010 12:01 AM

The only dead body I've ever seen that shouldn't have been dead was in a snow covered alley in Lewiston, Maine. I was covering a story 15 years ago about a man who'd been drinking who got into a fight with a man who'd been drinking, and one of them punched the other one and left him in the street overnight. The first man died of exposure.

The next day I got sent to cover the story and let me tell you I didn't want to go. Some reporter I was–half the time I wanted to help the people I was sent to get the interview from. The other half of the time I was wishing I'd called in sick–because murders, assaults, arsons–all of that made me sad. But the absolute worst– the sight of a dead man, or woman, or animal for that matter–made me ill. If I could have squeezed my eyes shut and stuck my fingers in my ears singing la-la-la-la-la-la until the whole thing was over, I would have. But it was my job to stay there and cover the story.

So I did it.

The only other dead bodies I've seen have been at wakes. I understand the religious purpose behind that and it makes many feel good to see and say good-bye to someone they love, but the first dead man I saw was my grandfather and I was 8 and I was petrified. He looked strange and not

human, deflated and flat lying there in the funeral parlor–
and at one point my elementary school imagination kicked
in and I swore he moved in the casket. I was freaked that
he'd sit up and yawn. I didn't sleep for days after that.

So I was reading a few of these anti-cancer books I've
bought recently to help me get a grip on what other things
I can do about this recurrence I'm in, when I got to a part I
hadn't read before. It said something like "and they were
twice as likely to reach the 5 year marker as those not
doing" blah blah blah. It wasn't the thing they were eating
that I focused on: it was the time frame. 5 years? That's
all?

Is that what "they" say I have left?

I know anything can happen. I know I don't have to be a
statistic. I know I can survive this with a lot of
information, education, hope, faith, medicine and family/
friends. I know that.

But let me say that in addition to all of those wonderful
reasons I plan to not be just a "twice as likely to reach"
cancer survivor is the fact that I do not plan to be lying,
sitting, standing or yawning in any casket any time soon.
Look, I've seen my share of dead bodies. I've seen them
frozen solid and I've seen them flat and lifeless and that's
not going to be me. I have way too much more life to live
for that.

So the next time I hear or read some time-ticking statistics about my "chances" of making it through this, I'll be the one with my eyes squeezed shut, fingers in my ears, humming la-la-la-la-la-la. Because regardless of the scary statistics and the breast cancer fear in my life, it's now my new job to hang in there and stay alive.

And I will do it.

FEAR ITSELF
Dec 8, 2010 09:35 PM

I have fought off the fear demon all day today, the day I got the news the Elizabeth Edwards, estranged wife of former vice-presidential candidate John Edwards, died yesterday of her recurrent breast cancer.

Some days are just like this.

I know what you're thinking–that her case and my case are nothing alike. Just because she got her diagnosis in 2004 and so did I; just because she had surgery, chemo and radiation like I did (though not the same kinds of them), and just because it returned like mine has, doesn't mean our cases are the same.

I know all that. Cerebrally, I do.

But honestly, this kind of thing is all it takes for this smart, strong, take-charge breast cancer person to have the emotional wind knocked straight out of her. I literally had to yoga breathe (remember lamaze class? *Breathe! 2-3-4.*) so I didn't hyperventilate during my day. Elizabeth Edwards couldn't make it. Oh God, what does that mean?

I am doing many different things in conjunction with traditional medicines to change my body so that the cancer in me can't survive. I am starving it, as I like to picture in my head, by cutting out sugar and dairy and taking supplements and eating whole grains, tons of veggies and fruits. I envision the little sucker getting smaller and smaller, like the witch melting in the Wizard of Oz after Dorothy soaks her with a bucket of water.

Still, the headlines of today have thrown what amounts to a bucket of liquid emotion on my beat-cancer enthusiasm—-fear. I know I won't be like her, I'm sure I won't be like her, but jeez, it's awfully scary–and I have to admit it.

And that's where I am right now–admitting some fear. That's an unfortunate part of this journey. I can't be Wonder Woman 7 days a week–every now and then the magic lasso twists around me and the truth comes out–today I am freaking terrified.

So I inhaled and exhaled my way through my Wednesday of Tension and wished it was this past weekend again, when Elizabeth Edwards wasn't dead and I was back kicking cancer's butt. Then I thought of what I did this weekend–I'd seen a local production of Annie with my kids. At one point the character of Franklin D. Roosevelt, facing the terror of the Great Depression, shouts out, "The only thing we have to fear is fear itself!" And as I *breathe!-2-3-4*'d my way to pick the kids up at school I realized the old politician was right. I was not fearing the cancer, I was fearing the fear of cancer. Now I just gotta do something about it.

Like I said, some days are just like this.

THE AVASTIN DEBATE
Dec 16, 2010 04:02 PM

Here's my problem with the Avastin debate–

it doesn't take into account the people for whom the drug works.

It's the same argument that in 2009 led the US Government Task Force to advise that women not have mammograms until they are fifty and to forget self breast exams all together. In studies the incidents of mortalities did not change with or without the exams, it said. Yet, that does little to shed light on the individuals for whom breast cancer self exams and mammograms are the reasons they are alive today–like me.

I remember watching Nancy Snyderman on the Today show when that bomb was dropped. She was in the hot seat trying to explain the seemingly outrageous advisement. She called the stories of hope, the ones where people could actually trace their lives back to an SBE or a mammogram, "anecdotal" stories. I'll never forget that–I know what she meant but all I could hear was that she called my life "anecdotal."

Sure I may not live as long as you will, but I know I am here today because 6 years ago during a self breast exam I felt a lump. My kids have memories of me that 6 years ago, at ages 4 and 1, they never would have had. Ask any psychologist the long term effect of a child losing a parent, and a mother specifically, at such a young age and they'll roll their eyes with that look of "it ain't pretty." And I know, my mother lost her mother when she was 8–not to breast cancer, to something else–but she's never been the same since.

There's a lot still to consider in this debate, most notably the cost of this drug–which is outrageous. And this country is in no position to dole out drugs that studies say do not produce the kind of results that make the debt worth it.

But out there are women who credit Avastin with giving them another day to hug their kids, check their email, see their next patient, or file that motion for dismissal. So if the FDA is now recommending to disapprove its usage for breast cancer patients, then I can assure you anyone interested in the incidence of "anecdotal" lives lost to this decision has a guaranteed study in the making on their hands.

Which means this is a sad day for sick people everywhere.

And I hope you never become one of us.

WHAT GETS ME THROUGH
Dec 18, 2010 06:57 PM

This week I had a down day. Goodness knows many others did too, I assume. Down days are a part of life and there's no real way to avoid them. You just have to get through them.

So in my down day I did what many others do--I tried to boost myself up. I watched a funny movie. I got a latte. I worked out with a dear friend--exercise AND support, the best! And above all I kept moving, moving through it--to the next place. Like Winston Churchill said, "When you're going through Hell, keep going."

Later in the day I got a call from a good friend. She wanted to get together. I thought about not responding, which is how I felt--I even let her phone call get picked up by the answering machine--I just didn't feel like talking. But honesty has always been my best policy and besides, I realized I wasn't afraid or ashamed of how I was feeling. It was just how I was feeling. So I emailed her and told her--I said I wasn't up for talking but I thanked her for reaching out. She emailed back saying she understood, and was here for me--and that made my dark day brighten a little.

And that's where I am today--grateful for the people who lighten my load with a quick email, a brief call, a text, a cup of tea, a voicemail, or a wave from a street corner as I drive by and see them biking their kids home from school.

Some days that's all I need--a whole bunch of those to make the blue day shift from navy to royal and then eventually--to bright sky blue.

My day ended with another good friend--a call just to say I'm thinking of you. The call barely lasted 2 minutes but the meaning and the sentiment went all all through my night--and into this morning. I am so grateful for my friends--or as I like to call them, my "people." Some days they are the one sure thing that gets me through.

BLIZZARD PERSPECTIVE
Dec 31, 2010 03:59 PM

I traveled this holiday and I got stuck in the blizzard of 2010 that blanketed the east coast of the United States, causing air flights to be cancelled from Bangor, Maine to Berkley, California. I was one of the lucky ones whose first flight got out on time--but I did have to stay overnight in a hotel in a state many states from my own in order to wait and hope that the next morning I would get back. And I did.

So I know people got stuck this holiday--I saw it first hand when I arrived at one mobbed airport and heard a woman shrieking at a travel agent "you've been lying to us all day!" And I know that it's so awful to sit in an airport with screaming kids or a sick aunt or no luggage or no snacks. And we all know how much I love spending five dollars on a bottle of airport water--NOT!

But as I sat there listening to that angry traveler ream out the ticket agent I couldn't help but think to myself, "I wish that was my biggest worry of the year--whether or not I'll be home tomorrow or the next day."

As someone battling recurrent breast cancer, I am terribly shaken by what may lie ahead. Will I be here to see my son graduate high school? Will I be able to help my daughter through her first heart break? Will I see 50 years? I just don't know.

Not to be completely detached from the mess and madness of lost suitcases, long lines and flights to nowhere, but as far as major life headaches go, I'd have traded places with any one of those upset folks in any of those airports this holiday season--in a heart beat.

THE "M" WORD
Jan 6, 2011 05:58 PM

There are a lot of words in the English language that are forbidden. They all have letters attached to them, letters like F (the "F" word) and C (the "C" word). Even L got mixed in there when the creators of a TV show on lesbianism thought they'd borrow the verboten connotation in order to grab attention and boost ratings. From what I hear it's a good show and many people watch so I think it worked–but technically the L Word is not in league with what I'm referring to.

I'm referring to those bad things that make us shudder; those words or visuals that are conjured up by throwing consonants and vowels together, breathing air into them, and using them to describe terrible things. The" S" word comes to mind–can't you just smell it?

So I'd like to add a new letter to the pile of F, C and S-word negative verbal phraseology: the M. And that's M for "the M word" whose definition, as I am now defining it, is metastatic. As in metastatic breast cancer.

Which I have.

Metastatic means that the cancer has traveled outside the original spot where it first appeared in a body. It means that after surgery, chemotherapy, radiation, lost hair, exhaustion, bleeding gums and missing an entire summer of my children's lives to battle back disease, a few rogue breast cancer cells beat the odds, hid out in my body and after 6 years have come out to wreak havoc once again in my system. They are now in the lining of my lung–outside the breasts, and–metastatically speaking–trying to kill me.

And that's the cold reality of this (insert F-ing word here) disease that I have and that is what I must face in 2011. There are no amount of letter words to describe how ticked off I am that this breast cancer thinks it has any right to be inside me right now. But I promise you that I am not going anywhere. You know me, I will do this. I'll use every letter in the alphabet if I have to but I will win, I will survive, I will beat the odds. I will. I will kick the S word out of this F-ing word M word's A word.

You have my word on that.

DEFINING A BAD DAY
Jan 11, 2011 12:56 AM

How do you know you're having a bad day?

For all of us in can be very different. You can run over broken glass in your car and blow a tire on the day your AAA runs out. You could cut loose a bunch of smaller clients in the morning to concentrate on your big money-making one, only to have her cut you loose at the end of the same day. You could pick up the phone when the bill collector calls for the eighth time–and he's calling from his cell phone outside your door.

Or you could be me, and finish picking lice out of your child's hair only to check your email and get a note from your doc confirming that your recurrent breast cancer tumor markers have gone up.

Honestly, some of my days are surreal. One minute I'm finding fruit-flies in my kiddo's toe head and the next I'm wondering if I'll be here for a next round of childhood domestic insect infestation. If I had a nit for every cancer cell swirling in my body and I could smother them in shampoo and a metal comb and be done with this personal plague I would be the happiest woman in the hair aisle of the pharmacy.

But that ain't gonna happen. So I close down my email, make an appointment to talk to my doctor, and hit the laundry room. There are two nasty things infiltrating our happy home: one of them will be smothered in hot water and special shampoo and be gone before I can say weekend.

The other one is just hanging in there, fighting back–a bad day waiting to happen again and again.

ARTS AND (CANCER) CRAFTS
Jan 15, 2011 10:32 PM

I usually don't do cancer-oriented classes. It's not that I see
no value in them-they help rejuvenate, orient, push people
toward or help them see a new goal in their lives–lives that
if anything like mine are confused, mixed up, what-the-
heck is going on with me cancer lives.

The reason I don't attend these things is that when I do I
always end up feeling like a cancer victim. I feel labeled,
the feel-sorry-for-her one, the poor slob who got hit with
incredible bad mojo.

So today it was unusual that I showed up at a cancer
"class"–a collage for the soul, as it was called. The point
was to get in touch with the things that make you–or me–
who I am. The topics were things like community and
council–but what it all boiled down to was who we were
amid our cancer crisis, and who we wanted to become
through it all.

At first I sat in the circle and got that get-me-outta-here
feeling as the leader of the group made her introductions. It
all sounded so pitiful, so "we want to help you unlucky
folks get through your rotten lives"–even though that's not
what she said. That's just what I heard.
Then it wast time for the 26 of us to get up and sift through
the dozens of pages in front of us and pick pictures that
represented us. The prompt was things that resonated with

the phrase "I am the one who..".. which is a little hokey for me–

but a part of me was already enjoying myself.

It's not that I loved being a cancer patient, or a qualifier for the free-to-cancer-people class, or had a burning desire to cut and paste. It was that I was able to return to my inner child whose favorite elementary school class was art and who in the middle of what could have been a busy Saturday at my 2-kids-a-husband-a-dog-a-pile-of-laundry-and-recurrent-breast-cancer home, I was sitting in a quiet room cutting out pictures and gluing them on a card, thinking about myself the entire time.

If you're like me, you never do that. You're always picking up someone else's coat, dishes, back pack, lunch box, and trying to figure out what's for dinner. It never ends. But today I was there, thinking about me, and not feeling the least bit guilty about it.

The reason I even accepted the invitation is because my dear friend Raychel invited me. Raychel is one of those people whom I love like a sister, but I never see her. We literally live 4 streets away from each other and I haven't seen her since the summer time. When she shot me an email asking if I wanted to attend this seminar, I replied in capitals YES. It could have been a nose picking contest for all I cared, I just wanted to see Raychel.

But as we sat next to each other giggling over what we were creating and realizing what it was revealing about ourselves to us and to the others in the room, I discovered I was having a great time.

And as I reached for a photo of a little boy goofing around with a kitchen pot over his head, it hit me that when the going gets tough for this cancer girl, there is strength to be found in stepping outside my comfort zone, giving new things a try and surrounding myself with a great friend, glue and a whole bunch of giggles.

WHAT FRIENDS CAN DO FOR ME

Jan 18, 2011 08:52 PM

A friend of mine recently emailed me and asked me how she could help me. It's been three months since I found out the breast cancer I fought off 6 years ago has come back, and she wished she could do something. She wasn't sure what something meant, she just wanted to help. Some way, any way.

I can imagine that feeling–the helplessness, the "what can I do" angst. Of course, unless you're a doctor with new meds or a researcher with a cure, there's not too much anyone can do for me. I'm in this one alone as far as the disease goes, and that is frustrating for my family and my friends–and this friend especially. I have many wonderful, wonderful friends and every one of them wants to "do something" for me.

I'm thinking it must be very hard to be my friend right now.

But here's a "something" that this friend has already done and is still doing now–as are all of my other friends: she's loving me through all this crap. Let me tell you there are days when I can't find a smile. There are times when I don't pick up the phone because I don't want to talk. There are moments, and they come without warning and come on like gang busters, when I am not me; instead I am a recluse, I am a loner, I am a fearful, frightened mess.

How's that for a BFF? Who'd ever sign up for that as their gal pal?

Yet through everything, my friends stick with me. They keep emailing, even if I don't respond. They keep calling even if I don't pick up. And with every text, voicemail and message, I am reassured that I am not alone.

That is the biggest "something" I can get right now.

There's a mess of worry and concern out there for this breast cancer fighter, and I thank my lucky stars every day for that. I love every one of my family and all my pals for that–that with all that's happening in their busy lives–jobs, kids, husbands, troubles–each one of them keeps my situation forefront in their minds and hearts, even though that comes with a price–the price of having a friend with cancer.

So what can you do for me?

I assure you–if you're my friend, you're already doing it.

MELTDOWNS AND MOVING ON
Jan 24, 2011 05:38 PM

I had a little meltdown recently and I couldn't get past it–a dark dreary feeling that I was losing my battle with cancer.

There's not much I can do about that kind of thing. In my recurrent breast cancer situation, I have to wait and see if I'll get better. There's no cause and effect, no hit and run, no drink this and feel better. They can't even cut out the cancer. It's gone "viral" so to speak–it's in little places all at once in my body. It's a new ballgame, not like my first go-round where the cancer cells were in neatly packaged tumors and the doctors could see them and take them out. With recurrence it's more complicated. The cells are "here" and "there" and they can't be grabbed and held. It's like shade on a lawn–it's there but you can't touch it. And you can't cut up the lawn and make it go away. You have to find out what's blocking the light up there and creating that shade in the first place, and then you have to kill it at its roots before it kills you.

How's that for a landscaping challenge?

That's what my doctors are up against. That's what all cancer doctors are up against. Because everyone's cancer "lawn" is kind of the same but at the same time very different: what might block light and cause dark shadows on my green grass may not do that on someone else's. All doctors can do is look at what's happened for other cancer patients and hope that the drugs they've got will work in my backyard to destroy whatever's trying to destroy me first.

Which is why I had this meltdown. I mean, I'm already living in this state of suspended belief–the one where I can't believe any of this is even real, never mind all these pharmaceutical drugs I have to ingest so my shaded lawn goes bright and green again––-and then some stranger last week told me she "felt bad" for me. We were talking and getting acquainted at this cancer conference and suddenly she blurted out– "I just feel so BAD for you!"

At first I laughed her off, like I try to do with all things stupid. But a few days later a dark cloud descended over me and within 24 hours I was on my couch with the doors locked not answering the phone, watching re-runs of Will and Grace to try to jump start my un-happy heart.

It took me a week and three seasons of Will and Grace but today I am back. I'm not proud of losing a whole week to fear but it happened, that's reality and I'm over it–at least for now. That's the way it goes on the cancer landscape: mostly sunny, sometimes cloudy, and some days I need a locked tent and a DVD season of comedy to weather the weather.

But that was yesterday. Today I'm moving on: I'm back outside, soaking up the sun, looking for a spade and a shovel and rooting around in my own backyard:

I've got some roots to kill.

STABILIZING WITH AN "I"
Jan 29, 2011 08:21 PM

Good news: my doctors says my tumor markers are STABILIZING! Finally – something going my way in this fight against recurrent breast cancer!

I was so excited when I got this news I almost exploded. It's not like my doc told me the cancer had gone away, or that they'd found a cure, or that this was all a bad dream and I was really a healthy woman with young kids and a bright future. Yet for as excited as I got when I read her email, she might as well have told me all that. I was elated and couldn't wait to tell the world.

I got right on email and shot off a fast note to my family and some friends to let them in on what I'd been told; the good, great news that the medicine I'm taking to beat down cancer is working! But in my excitement–and my hope for dramatic flair by spelling out stabilizing with dashes–aka S-T-A-....I accidentally spelled the word incorrectly, so instead of saying "the tumor markers are S-T-A-B-I-L-I-Z-I-N-G with an I, I wrote S-T-A-B-A-L-I-Z-I-N-G with an A.

Being a writer and a news journalist by trade, making spelling errors is a big deal. And being a television news journalist is even worse as you have to know how to say AND spell everything (I remember once being made fun of by my executive producer for pronouncing indictment with a hard 'C'.) But I'm not a TV reporter any more, and specifically at this moment I wasn't reporting or even working– I was doing emotional jigs in my living room that my future was turning around and that I may live longer than these last few months have seemed possible. Which is good for the bright-future department of my life but apparently a lousy dictionary moment for me.

I got many positive feedback emails from family and friends, wishing me well, telling me they love me, and rooting me on. How many of them realized I'd spelled stabilizing wrong I don't know–because no one said anything–except one person. And that one person is a friend and family member who said he "couldn't resist" pointing out to me the spelling error–just to be a wise guy. Which is fine with me because we have that kind of relationship and I know he loves me and has my back.

But in case you got that original email, I want you to know I will never again make the mistake of misspelling stabilizing. The word is like music to my cancer fighting ears, and if I ever have to ask myself if there's an a or not in the word, I'll just remember the "I"–as in I am stabilizing these tumor markers!

As for the hard C in indictment, let me just say I never have had an indictment so why would I know how to spell it? And it should be a GH anyway–if we light and we fight, why don't we indight?.

But that's another blog for another day. Today I'm focused on the I in stabilizing and how I plan to fight (with a GH) and win–also with an I!– this battle with breast cancer.

ENOUGH WITH THE TIGER MOM
Jan 31, 2011 01:38 PM

In reading a friend's blog titled 'Extreme Parenting: East Vs. West, in which she discussed author Amy Chua's book, "Tiger Moms" and whether or not her readers parented "east" (Chua's way) or "west" (Americana-Dr. Sears-Helicopter style.) I'd like to chime in and say this:

When you think you may be dying, none of this crap matters. Whether Amy Chua or Oprah or Dr. Spock or Dr. Sears agrees with you, how you raise your child is your business. As in: trust your instincts, your experience, your friends that you admire and the children you hope your kids turn out like. Find out what worked there and morph it into what works in your own living room--not what works in some distanced country 6 thousand miles away.

I am so very tired of bookstores and talk show guests making me and you feel like we don't know how to do a job that 200 years ago everybody had to figure out on their own. You may have asked your local preacher or your auntie or your governess for help--not every single person who just tweeted their new formula for mommy success or the 300 titles stacked neatly in a row at Borders or Amazon.com's pediatric growth and development section.

I say enough already--parenthood doesn't come with a sticker price and a road map. Figure it out and love your kids on your own--

while you're still lucky enough to be here to do it.

I NEED YOUR HELP
Feb 9, 2011 08:13 AM

I need surgery this week. Surprised? Join the club.

It seems the breast cancer, which whose tumor markers were stabilizing–with an 'i'--has somehow managed to take over one of my lungs. I need to go have it drained and burned–yep, I just put 'lung' and 'burn' in the same sentence–so that this freaking disease has a harder time getting in.

As I like to ask to lighten the mood, "how we doing?"

Seriously, this is just insane. But so is the cancer ride. Like my first go-round with this insidious disease, it's one step forward, two steps back–and this week it's two steps way WAY back.

I'll be in the hospital for three days beginning Friday, and then home hopefully in time for my husband to shower me with Godiva chocolates on Valentine's Day. And since my lung has just been burned, if he doesn't I will breathe fire at him until he gets his sweet buns out the door to the nearest high-end confectionery and gets this girl what she wants after a long day (weekend) at the cancer office.

Here's what I need you:

This Friday at 4 o'clock Eastern Time, 3 o'clock Central Time, 2 o'clock Mountain Time and 1 o'clock Pacific Time I need you to stop what you're doing and think of me. I just need a minute of your mind space to send me some good vibes. When I first did this–when I went through double mastectomy surgery 7 years ago–I asked my friends to do this and it worked. I was beyond calm when I went under the knife. No pill, placebo or anesthetic has ever had that kind of effect on me.

This time I am hoping you'll do it for me again–hold my hand so to speak out in cyberspace so that I remember that through this procedure–and through this metastatic hell–I am not alone.

Thank you.

GET YOUR CLAPPING HANDS READY
Feb 17, 2011 05:28 PM

I wanted to let you all know the results of my operation. The surgery itself seems like a success– I am at home, breathing well on two functioning lungs and able to walk at least 10 minutes a day. Tomorrow I plan to make it 20.

The information from my surgery is less than elevating. It seems I have more cancer in my body than previously realized. I'll start chemotherapy in 2 weeks to knock it down and then get back on hormone therapy to keep the breast cancer beast at bay–for what I plan to be many many years to come.

So how am I doing with all this? I'm mad as hell.

This is unacceptable. I can not believe that this disease thinks it has any right in my body, never mind flourishing in it. I have so much to do in my future, so much of my life's gift still to give. No damn disease is going to stop me.

So with help from my doctors, my family and from my friends–pharmaceutical and otherwise–I will do whatever it takes to win against cancer. But I have to admit right now I'm not feeling so strong.

Where I live it is raining today and if the weather were a mirror on my feelings this would be the perfect reflection.

I look up at the soaking clouds and feel solidarity with the skyline–because I'm soaking too, on the inside. I am sick of being sick and I am tired of being tired. I am so not the type for this role I'm playing–and I want OFF THIS SET.

But here's the thing, I can't bail. I can't walk off. That would be curtains for sure. The cancer would win. So I know I must go on. I get that. I also get that this whole thing is happening to me but it's not all about me. There's other stuff, stuff I don't understand. I have no clue–why me, why now, why breast cancer, why isn't it stopping, and why did it have to rain today? Today, 3 days from my release from hospital after they sucked 2 pints of fluid off my left lung and I just want to walk in the sunshine and heal? Why is that too much to ask?

And while we're at it, why have I never liked to cook, why did I just eat 2 boxes of Godiva chocolates all by myself, and why do I sound like a skater from the 1994 Winter Olympics who just had a bat put to her ankle? Why? Good Lord, what is going on here?

I have no freaking idea. I just don't. And apparently, I'm not going to find out today. What I do know is this: I have to keep moving, keep reading the cancer script as the pages fall in front of me–some of them blank and most of them gibberish–and take this show on the chemo road–AGAIN.

I have no idea how long this Cancer Charade will run but I'll tell you one thing, the show will not close early. If this is some kind of big moment I will make it worth your time and my price of admission. I will ROCK THIS STAGE. And I will be around for many, many ovations.

So get your clapping hands ready.

MOTIVATE

Motivation is hard to find in my life this week–which I've already told you.

And today, having broken the news to our children about upping my cancer battle game with chemotherapy in a few weeks, motivation is even harder. People may think "don't your kids' faces motivate you enough?" and I can honestly say "yes–and no." Yes because they need me and I want to live to help guide them in their futures. But no in the sense that inadvertently dragging them through this truly breaks my heart. When she should be worrying about when that next play date will be and he should be more concerned with what kind of 12th birthday party he should plan, they're worrying about losing me. What kid deserves that?

So when I opened an email from my brother-in-law this week I got an unexpected boost. Stephen is an athlete and he's been running, biking, hiking and freewheeling his way around the country with his wife for decades. If there's a mountain in the way, Stephen climbs it–literally. His reasons for doing so are always those that a non-athlete like me doesn't understand: because I can.

Today he's doing this crazy 24 hour bike ride–one that you don't sleep through. I have to state that because although it seems obvious to not sleep through a day long bike ride I just have to repeat it. He doesn't S-L-E-E-P. Not only that but he BIKES the whole time. It's like a college all-nighter, minus the coffee and Doritos, add a bike and ride it from college campus to the next state or 200 miles–whichever comes first. But for Stephen–and this is unusual for him–he was having trouble finding his motivation. He writes,

"I considered raising money for some worthy cause – kids, Africa, Bangladesh, Haiti,.. – but I couldn't raise enough determination to ask all my friends and family for money for something that was ultimately serving to motivate me to ride my bike … (But) tonight..I found myself getting stoked all over again for the ride. And I know in large part I have you to thank… Your battle has been a wonder to watch. Your determination, hope, attitude – despite the underlying unknowns and easy access to doubt – have put me in the best frame of mind I could possibly ask for for this insignificant undertaking."

I've been a mother, a wife, a daughter, a sister, an aunt, a (lousy) godmother, and a friend: but I've never been a motivation for an athlete before. I have to tell you, it feels pretty good.
He sent me a photo of himself and his bike–and taped to the front is my picture. He finishes his email saying,

"You and I have our own races going on. Mine's shorter and way easier. But you and I will go through them together."

So while I struggle to find my motivation to get through my future, today I'll also be doing laps on the front of a racing bike with the breeze blowing through my inkjet-printed hair hanging on for dear life and pushing my bro-in-law Stephen through his paces to find his motivation to win his battle, too.

Wish us both luck.

TICKET TO RIDE
Feb 23, 2011 12:14 PM

Do you like amusement parks? Or more specifically, do you like roller coaster rides?

Grab a handrail and read on, because if I'm not on the biggest loop-de-loop of a life I don't know what I'm on...

I got amazingly GREAT news from my oncologist yesterday. This is the same oncologist who, like my lung oncologist after my surgery last week, saw all kinds of cancer in my pulmonary region and thought "Oh sh-t, this girl needs chemo."

But three days ago, my tumor markers came back—the ones that had been stabilizing a month ago and then faked me out when all this cancer was found—and are reading not just stable but DROPPING. And not just dropping a few percentage points but really plunging downward, in one case by almost 50 percent!

Did you lose your breath? Join the club. As my sister-cousin said to me yesterday when she got this latest news, "I don't think we're tall enough to be on this ride!" (She lives near Disneyland.)

Seriously, this is nuts. One day we're up, one day we're down. Yesterday I'm preparing my kids for a hairless, exhausted shell of a mother and today I'm dancing toward them with their breakfast plates full of food I just cooked because I had the energy–and the hope–that goes along with good news.

How'd it happen? It's hard for a non-medical person to explain it, but the doctors said something like: the cancer they found, which on first blush looked like new cancer, is really likely old cancer that they hadn't realized was there. And part of the reason they hadn't realized it is because I look, act and am trying to be as healthy, active and as upbeat as I can. In other words, I don't act like a cancer 'patient'–if there is a definition to that, and I'm not sure there is. We patients go through a whole load of junk on this journey and who we are changes and morphs every which way through out the experience. I don't recommend a ticket to this ride.

But for now, I have to thank you for helping me out. I know this is exhausting for you as well as for me, and as my husband asked me last night, "Do you think we'll suffer from 'friend fatigue'? Do you think at some point our friends are just gonna bow out because this is all too much for them?" I thought about that for a second; certainly that could happen. Hell I'm fatigued and it's happening to me. If I could step off this ridiculous ride I would, so why not you?

So I figure this: if you need to bow out for awhile and get some popcorn, a drink and a long walk far away from this Spacey Mountain, you go right ahead. We will not hold

that against you. (And if you could some day take my
husband with you and buy him a
beer(s) so he could forget about this for a nano-second, I'll
buy the drinks.)

This is a ride I'll be on for the rest of my life, and I don't
expect any of you to hang on to every twist, lift and
plummet. I really don't.

But I do want you to be there when this terrifying machine
has slowed down and I can unclench the handrail and catch
my breath--vibrant, healthy, and tall enough to have
withstood the ride.

RADIATION RAY, PART ONE
Feb 26, 2011 04:59 PM

One of the questions I get asked from an audience every time I speak about my film *The Breast Cancer Diaries* is this: "Was there anything in the film that you couldn't include that you wish you could have?"

My joking answer is, "Yes–there's about 7 extra seconds of my husband walking in front of my diary camera in his boxer shorts that I wanted to keep, but for time sake we had to cut." After the laughter, I usually say, "No, it's all in there."

That is until this week, when a dozen whoopie pies--that New England cake and cream filled delicacy--arrived at my doorstep and I remembered that there was an entire story line that did not make air.

Let me back up:

In 2004, after my bilateral mastectomy and 8 rounds of dose-dense chemotherapy, I had 25 rounds of radiation to go before my breast cancer treatments were over. When I arrived at the Bath, ME facility to start the zapping, I was scared.

This tall, affable, lovely man named Ray told me he would be my radiation technician. That means he'd help me up onto the long flat table, bind my feet so I didn't move, and close the big, metal door that said "DANGER: KEEP OUT" separating me, on the wrong side of the danger door, from the outside world that did not have cancer.

He'd also come back inside the room in between the 3 radiation hits to make sure I hadn't moved–so that the invisible beams were hitting the exact right spots to hopefully keep my cancer from ever coming back. I was still scared but Ray–or Radiation Ray as I kiddingly started to call him–was so kind that he made me feel better every time I went.

When you have that kind of a close (every day) but brief (the treatments lasted 10 minutes tops) relationship with someone, even a stranger, you talk. And you bond. I told Ray about my kids, my husband, my love of whoopie pies, and that I freelanced at Maine PBS. He told me the sometimes-receptionist at the radiation front desk was his wife, that they lived in a darling old home on a hill in Bath, and that he often worked behind the scenes at the local "Chocolate Church" production house.

Over the 6 weeks we saw each other about a half an hour every week day, and I really began to see Ray not just as a technician but as a friend.

And it was with that kind of friend-to-friend excitement that I came into radiation one day toward the end of my treatments and told Ray that I was getting back to work at PBS. I was doing a show that night in fact, and since I hadn't had the energy or strength to work since my diagnosis 6 months earlier I was very excited–and nervous, too–to "get back on the horse" as they say. I was going to be normal again, if only for one night.

Ray was thrilled for me! He promised that he and his wife Nancy would watch. He'd put sticky notes up so as not to forget–and we'd talk about the show the next day when I came in for my regularly scheduled radiation.

That night I did the show, I went on air again. Seeing HOST, ANN MURRAY, as the credits rolled was a much needed boost for my cancer-weary soul. With a wig and professional make-up I'd anchored an hour long civic affairs program on education in the state of Maine. It went off without a hitch–I even threw off my fake breasts 10 minutes to air and said "let it be!" and no one noticed the difference–and I couldn't wait to ask Ray what he thought. Could he believe that skinny, sick patient he strapped onto his radiation table each day was the same strong anchor woman who nailed that PBS show the night before?

The film's director (and my sister-in-law and friend) Linda Pattillo and I went into the office the next day with the camera rolling. Ray met us at the entrance to the treatment area and I smiled a wide smile. "Did you watch the show?" I grinned. "Yes I did!" Ray beamed. And then he said,

"You know, I met Ann Murray once. She was always my favorite when she worked at WCSH6."

I stood there, confused. Surely he was kidding. I was Ann Murray. What did he mean by that?

TO BE CONTINUED

RADIATION RAY, PART TWO
Feb 27, 2011 02:43 PM

THIS IS PART TWO OF A THREE PART BLOG.

And Ray went on:

"I met her once at Kristina's Restaurant. She was having lunch just before she had her baby and she hadn't been on TV at Channel 6 forever. And I stopped over and even though my wife didn't want me to bother her, I had to tell her that she was my favorite news reporter and I couldn't wait to have her come back after her maternity leave."

I stood there, completely lost. What was he talking about?

And then it hit me like a key light falling from the rafters on a well-lit television set. I remembered that guy. I remember the fan who'd stopped by my table as I shoved a hefty caesar salad into my pregnant stomach and prayed that my water would break so I could have my body back. I remember him saying how he loved to see me out on the sidewalks in a snowstorm with my big suede hat, telling people that it was, in fact, snowing. I looked at tall, affable Ray and realized--this is THAT guy!

And then--*oh my word he has no idea who I am.*

He has NO IDEA that Ann the savvy television anchor he adored and Ann the sick cancer patient he sees every week day of the week (and likely pities every night when he and Nancy go home after work) are ONE AND THE SAME person.

AND--he has no idea that that was me last night anchoring that live PBS show either. He thinks I was working on the show-- behind the scenes.

Linda had the camera rolling, picking up every sound--but the silence was deafening. I still just stood there. My mind was racing.

And then I knew why he didn't know me. I'd never talked about my former TV job while strapped to the radiation table. It was too many worlds away from what I was in the middle of now with this beating-back-cancer diagnosis. And being a tiny, gray-skinned, hairless and breast-less cancer patient, I in no way resembled the bold TV reporter who'd used her bilingual skills to help blow the lid off the Decoster Egg Farm-migrant worker scandal in Turner a few years back, or celebrated the comeback of the Androscoggin River every spring.

And because I came into the office registered with my married name, Ann Paige, not Ann Murray, my television name, Ray would never have made the connection that I was actually Ann MURRAY Paige, former NBC StormCenter queen and Lewiston Bureau turned anchor reporter who left WCSH6 after she had her baby and turned up hosting civic affairs programs on Maine PBS for the last 6 years....including last night.

Oh my word. How weird is THIS? And....*what do I do now?*

RADIATION RAY, THE FINALE
Feb 28, 2011 02:46 PM

THIS IS THE LAST IN A SERIES OF THREE BLOGS.

I stood there, still unsure of what to say--but pretty clear now on what had happened, and pretty clear on what was about to happen.

Ray didn't know who I was, and I had to tell him.

I felt bad--bad for Ray that he didn't know who I was and that once I told him it might be embarrassing. And fighting off a creeping sorry-for-myself feeling, too. I mean, did I really look THAT bad?

"Ray," I said, coming out of my growing pity party to focus on the tall, sweet gentleman who'd been so good and kind to me these last 5 weeks (this really was turning into the king of all awkward moments,)

"Ray, I *AM* Ann Murray."

Dead silence. Now it was his turn to be confused.

The entire moment--as well as the minutes afterward when I explained it all to Ray--were caught on film, and Linda and I have those tapes in a safety deposit box with the rest of the 100 mini-DV films taped during the making of *The Breast Cancer Diaries*. Unfortunately, like the back story before it, it was impossible to weave the tale of Ann the Anchor and Radiation Ray into the film. It was too far removed from the main story of Ann beating cancer's butt and getting back on the horse of her life.

But the relationship that I have with Ray is now stronger than ever. The stories we have together, begun in the radiation room and prequel-ed with the whole "I met Ann Murray once" flashback have made us lifelong friends.

In fact, on the day I finished my last radiation back in 2004, I went out to my car and found half a dozen whoopie pies nestled in a pink box on the hood of my car. "Not all at once, okay?" was the note from Ray and his wife--also my new friend--Nancy. I burst into tears. Just like I did this week, 7 years later, when the UPS man delivered a full dozen Wicked Whoopie Pies to my door. "A little bit of home for you" was the note from Ray and Nancy.

Which is why the next time somebody in an audience asks me if there's something that happened during the filming of The Breast Cancer Diaries movie that we had to cut that I wish we could have left in, along with my husband's 7 seconds of skin, I'll say,

"Yes. Radiation Ray."

WORDS WITH FRIENDS
Mar 4, 2011 01:05 PM

My cousin Sarah, whom I consider a sister, got me into the game "Words with Friends" on the Iphone. Basically it's Scrabble long distance. She and I "play" hundreds of miles away from each other and our phones both ding when one of us has created a word and it's the other's turn.

I got into it during her last visit to see me, when chemotherapy was looming on my cancer horizon and she, as usual, had come up to help. Part of helping was engaging me in this thinking game and giving us yet another connection to each other when she eventually had to hop a flight and return home to her real life. Of course, she'll be back, she always comes back–but "Words" keeps up together daily with our double letter and triple word score connection.

This week I lost yet another game to her–she is the consummate wordsmith–(did you know that QI is a word?)–but as I began another game with her, my son and I were sitting on the couch talking about how I don't have to start chemo this week. He is so happy, so relieved, and we were doing a little dance around the house and humming "no chemo, no chemo" when he came asked me, "When you don't have to have chemotherapy, what's it called?" And before I could answer, he took a shot at it: "unchemo?"

I laughed out loud–YES! And I gave him the greatest hug a metastatic mom has ever given her pre-pubescent, eyes-as-big-as-saucers, sweetheart of a scared son. "Unchemo! That's it!"

So I'm just warning you, Sarah, that if in our next game of Words I put down a 6 letter word that gets me 22 points because I'm on a double word square, and that words starts with a U and ends with an O, but you've never heard of this word–it's a real word. And it means relief.

LUCKY ME
Mar 5, 2011 04:44 PM

Three weeks ago today I was sitting in a hospital bed with two feet of tubes stuck up my left lung trying to avoid asphyxiation by breast cancer. Today I walked a 7K. Guess who's feeling lucky?

And the name of this 7K as Irish luck would have it is the "Lucky 7". And I was feeling pretty fortunate–- not just because it was partly sunny and 65 degrees (this run BTW NOT in Maine!) perfect weather for an athletic event. And not just because the name, Lucky 7, contains my favorite number, seven. Not even because I had my husband by my side as we high tailed it down the path, passing a few people but watching many serious athletes fly by us, in search of a win, a second, or maybe a tie–while all we worried about was what flavor gatorade we'd get at the next refreshment station.

I didn't feel lucky for any one of these reasons I just listed but for every one of them. Three weeks ago I couldn't get out of bed without two machines dragging behind me and the threat of a bed pan if I didn't. I would have cracked a shillelagh over anyone's head who tried to make me walk the surgery floor much less strap on Nikes and beat feet for an hour and ten minutes through a city.

But today was different. On this day I geared up, headed out, hit the roadways and practically did the Irish jig as I sailed through my 7K, 3 weeks post surgery. Breast cancer ain't gonna get the best of this shamrock. And rainbows and a pot of gold to my cracker jack surgical team for doing such a great job that all I have to show for my ordeal are three scabs and a hint of hospital tape residue.

I was determined upon leaving the hospital this past Valentine's Day that for this upcoming Irish sweat event I would be ready to go. And I feel so fortunate that I was. I am grateful to the non-profit for putting on the run and I was thrilled that my husband decided last minute to join me. As we walked and watched the Ks go by, I couldn't help but feel like I was kickin' some cancer butt as I did.

So that was my day. I did the Lucky 7. Or as I like to think of it now, the *Lucky Me*.

CANCER HOROSCOPE
Mar 8, 2011 12:35 PM

I logged into my Facebook account and saw a friend's post of her Daily Cancer Horoscope. I got a quick punch-in-the-gut feeling when I saw it, thinking she was announcing that she has cancer. Then I realized she was born in July and it was a real "this is what's in the stars for you today" entry. My stomach unclenched and I moved on to see what other friends were up to today.

But it has stayed with me. I've been thinking of my own present cancer horoscope. If there was a site I could go to that would tell me what the cards held for me today I wonder what it would say. Something like, " today your tumor markers are receding: it's the perfect day to kick some cancer butt."

I got online at horoscope.com, looked at today's entry, and read it. It is positive, full of possibilities, and frankly kind of obvious. It could be anybody's horoscope–even mine. But I have metastatic breast cancer, so the lessons of a horoscope need a little tweaking in order to really be something I can relate to.

So I decided to add a little dimension to the stars today-- and this is it: I call it Cancer Horoscope , *The Medical Edition.*If you're in my same boat– fighting cancer and hoping like hell you're winning–I'm right there with you. And this blog's for you.

Cancer Horoscope: The Medical Edition

Start something new after lunch when the Moon settles in Taurus. *Jupiter, Saturn, who cares– just do it. Time is of the essence. So what if you fail, just start.*

If you're single, a romance that starts tonight could become a solid relationship. *And if you don't feel a sizzle, it's a fizzle–MOVE ON. Heaven knows you're going through enough without a lame partner dragging you down.*

You and your significant other realize how snap judgments cause problems. *Forget the snap–judgements blow altogether. Focus on understanding. Find common ground. He's doing his best, and so are you.*

Never underestimate the power of the words "I'm sorry"– *and expect to hear them back, too. You deserve forgiveness as much as you give it.*

Finish unfinished business. *While you're still here to do it.*

THE SURPRISE
Mar 15, 2011 11:25 AM

This past weekend marked an important day for me–the anniversary of my breast cancer diagnosis. I do something special this time of year to celebrate the life I still have.

I've gone to inns and hotels, broadway and beaches with girlfriends, with my family, with my husband, with people who are close. And close by. Because when you live far from the ones you love your opportunities to share celebrations can be few and far between.

Which brings me to my surprise. I didn't want to chance that anyone whom I'm about to sneak up on would read about it before I had a chance to pull it off. But now that I did it, I can spill the beans.

The back story is: I have a godmother whom I adore. Like my mother did, Darlin gave me guidance and strength, love and belief in myself from the day she held me in that white gown on the christening altar until this very day. As an insecure child then, I needed it. As a sick adult today, I cherish it.

What she's meant to me my entire life is impossible to blog because the blog would fall into cyberspace with the emotional weight of her importance to me. Suffice to say she's as close to my mother in terms of shaping the woman

I've become than any other human being save my own mother herself. (And that's another blog altogether.)

And Darlin is old. I don't think she'll be mad at me for saying that because when you reach 90, age flows through that middle age horror place through the retirement year wrinkle phase to a place I assume is like reaching Mount Everest: The I Did It Place. As in: I'm still here, attending my grandchild's wedding, holding my great-grandchildren in my arms, loving the children I have, and the godchild.

Which is me.

So I flew across the country to surprise her on her 90th birthday weekend, which was this past weekend. And it's been a bit of a nail biter for me because four weeks ago my breast cancer landed me in emergency surgery with tubes in my lung and a 4 week embargo on flying.

Meanwhile Darlin has her own lung issues. Breathing is difficult when you've hit your 9th decade and her own air space is not so clear. We have both been fighting for oxygen recently and let me say the irony is not lost on me.

But I got my all clear to fly from my doc last Tuesday and arranged a secret trip (and yes I bought flight insurance. For me these days, a must.)

And this past Friday night, I stood on Darlin's doorstep, 3-thousand miles from where she thought I'd be. To see her face when I walked through the door was worth all the travel, the money, the health hassle and the nail biting. Within minutes we were holding glasses of chardonnay, laughing and hugging and holding onto our moment. That's what celebrations of life are all about. And if ever there was a double reason to celebrate life, her 90th and my any-th are the reasons to do it.

I have many people to thank for making me who I am today, and this weekend I got to help blow out 90 candles on one of those person's birthday cake. It's been an honor to have my godmother in my life and this past weekend, it was an honor to celebrate her life–right by her side.

Happy Birthday, Darlin. I love you.

MY DAD'S DEMENTIA
March 15, 2011 04:33 PM

My Dad has dementia. Maybe yours does too. If he does you know the look I'm about to talk about, the one where his eyes look at you but they aren't quite sure who they're looking at.

My Dad and I had a strained relationship as I grew up. He was hard on me and I was hard on me so I learned to fear him and be afraid of me. Or rather, be afraid to try to be me. Instead I behaved the way I thought he and my mother wanted me to, and as a result took a long time to discover who Ann really was. Along the way, some dreams were lost. I'm sure many reading this blog have a similar story, as parents are not perfect.

Today, however, my father is perfect. Not mentally–mentally he's quite imperfect. The doctors say his dementia is caused by wounds he received in World War 2. It's a hell of a delayed price to pay for putting your life on the line for your country, and a protracted price to pay for freedom. But because of this wounded way of getting the disease, Dad's dementia plays out in the most unusual way: he is a love.

And growing up I could never have described my dad that way. I was afraid of him. He was a nice man–respectable, honest, sincere and hardworking. But as the son of a doctor from Boston and the 7th of 8 children, my father was not the warm and fuzzy type. I don't remember him ever reading me a book, holding my hand or telling me he loved me.

Of course he did love me. He took incredibly great care of me and my sisters and brother. We all have college degrees, we all had a roof over our head, private schools and bicycles. He did well by us, and we learned honesty, integrity and character from him.

But we didn't learn hugs and kisses–until now.

Now my father, in his demented state, can't stop telling me how good I look. He may not remember my name but he sure as hell takes every opportunity to tell me my teeth are gorgeous, my hair looks great and that my pajamas make me look like a movie star.

When he comes down in the morning for breakfast Dad sings my mother's name with a childlike quality that would make a preschooler giggle. He kisses her three times on the forehead goodnight as he pats her freshly coifed head and tells her how amazing her hair looks, how wonderful she is.

And he is never at a loss to tell me how he'd be lost without her. "She's so good to me," he purrs, and she is. In 2012 they will be married 60 years and these last 4 years my mother has strained under the "for worse" clause more than she expected she'd have to. Having a husband who used to rule the roost now cling to you for toothbrushing instruction is a mind-blower at any age, never mind the so-called golden one.

But both she and I know it could be much "worse" than the "for worse" she's dealing with. So we attempt to count our blessings. Fighting metastatic breast cancer makes me search for the positives more now than ever, and mom's in a similar boat. After all, what other choice do we have?

I'll never know what it's like to watch the man I married 58 years ago strain to follow a sentence. Or forget the day. The date. The name of his son. How to turn on a radio.

But I do know two things: to have my father tell me he loves me more times than I can count in a day is a gift I will gratefully accept with an open if not breaking heart. And to have a mother put one foot in front of herself each day and try her best while facing her "worst", even when her best doesn't quite reach the mark she'd hoped for, is a lesson in courage, honor and grace that I hope I live up to,

whatever the 'worst' that may still await me.

OUT OF CONTROL
Mar 16, 2011 09:28 AM

I was watching the news with my mother this morning about the Japanese earthquake. What horrible devastation, what trauma, what fear–not only for the Japanese but for all of us. It was all so out of control. Watching their lives wash away from thousands of miles away I got that sinking feeling– what if that happened to me?

Then the morning program did what I hate–the "are you prepared for your dose of devastation" story. They talked about my town's potential lack of disaster plan, lack of water, lack of resources, lack of lack. It was such a downer that I had to walk out of the room. I felt anxious and scared and I hadn't even gotten out of my pajamas. At this rate, lunchtime could pose a serious threat to my nervous system.

And it got me thinking–while being prepared is important in all regards, being uber-prepared for everything can be paralyzing. So far in my life I've been warned about nuclear war, terrorism attacks, plagues, pandemics, cancer, heart attacks, alcohol poisoning, sun spots, liver damage, vitamin B12 deficiency, stroke, bad breath, broccoli in my teeth, panty lines, hot flashes, cold sweats, hangovers and hang nails. I could go on but you've got grocery shopping and kids to pick up.

Here's all I'm saying: some things will be out of our control. As much as we strive to avoid what is billed as something we can avoid if only we do blah blah blah, the truth is stuff happens in life. And as much as we can prepare, something is bound to get us.

So live your life well, have faith in your faith, give to others and take good care of yourself. Prepare as well as you can and then let it be. Despite what the articles and news story say, much of what's going to happen to us is out of our control.

And if anything bad does happen to me–which it has with my breast cancer–I just remember one thing: I'm doing my best. And ultimately, that's the only real thing I truly can control.

ICE CREAM AND ENVY
Mar 28, 2011 04:45 PM

One of the hardest things for me about being a cancer patient--aka fighter, survivor-back-battling-again, or whatever you are when you have metastatic breast cancer-- is what other people go through around me.

I'm talking about the strange syndrome that I don't know if it has a name but I'll try to describe it. It's the feeling that I, as the cancer patient, am receiving nice things, heaped-on attention, and have so much sympathy thrown my way that sometimes those around me can begin to feel, for lack of a better word, jealous of me.

The supreme irony being that who in the world is truly jealous of a cancer patient? Nobody is.

But I actually understand and appreciate the validity of this syndrome because it happened in my first go-round with breast cancer. When I was getting unexpected visits from dear friends from miles away and having whoopie pies delivered to my door, some in my life were feeling like Santa forgot to fill their stockings, too. And the people closest to me began to feel left out-- not of the cancer of course, but of the attention I was getting.

There's no easy way to get around this syndrome--which emulates survivor guilt but is more like survivor envy--at least I haven't found a way around it. And maybe you haven't, either. After all, when anything bad happens to friends or even strangers, we-- the ones who don't experience the trauma--often rush to the side of the person, or give money, or donate-- because we want to show our love and compassion. And maybe there's even a little bit of a verboten sense of relief that it's not happening to us going on in there too--I don't know. Whatever it is, I think it's all normal.

But the abnormal creeps in when we're the ones watching all this goodness literally happen around us and we--in our imperfect human forms-- want a little for ourselves. It's like the kid next to you getting a second helping of ice cream because his dropped. Meanwhile yours is all gone because you ate yours--yet you still feel a little jealous of Mr. I-still-have-a-fresh-new-cone. Like I said, I think it's all normal.

I don't know what to say about this syndrome except that, like all things cancer, it sucks.

And if you're feeling this syndrome, I promise you, I understand--and I sure don't hold it against you.

But if you ever need some help getting by it, just know this: the good stuff I get is far outweighed by the bad feelings I stuff deep down inside me every day about my future. Things like the doctors telling me that eventually ones cancer gets so used to the meds it begins to outsmart them--and take over. Or the fear I feel each time I go into an infusion room and see people curled up in recliners with IVs in their arms, crying. Or the skeletal photos of Dennis Hopper before he died of cancer.

All that crap–the fear of physical pain, emotional suffering, shriveling illness and a premature death—-I feel it all the time. Of course I don't live in that space day to day or I'd go insane, but these feelings are always on my perimeter, and I can't push then away because they are the realities of my cancer life.

I know you love me and that what you sometimes feel about my cancer swag is a natural feeling--so go ahead and feel it. Just know that if I could give up this second helping of ice cream that's being forced down my throat and never lick this friggin cone again, I would.

MY COUSIN SARAH
Mar 29, 2011 09:29 PM

I had a cousin when I was little named Sarah. We lived 8 states away from each other, saw the other rarely if ever, and never spoke on the phone. We were a year and a day apart in age and worlds away from each other in gifts–she a tomboy, spoke her mind, unafraid to defend herself in a fight; me a Lipsmacker lover, cautious and worried, and always afraid to defend myself in a fight.

Yet somehow, every time I saw her–at the occasional wedding, catholic holiday or old relative funeral, was like was coming back to the pool after too long in the sun —"aaaaahhhhhh." She was one of my dearest friends and though I had 4 of them at home I saw Sarah as a sister. My sister. And any time we were together, I knew I was going to have a blast.

Then we grew up. Time took us traveling–she moved a few times, we both went to high school, then college and graduate schools and then off to big cities and new friends. Throw in our respective climbs up the career ladder–hers in marketing and mine in TV journalism, and a romantic relationship or two and we lost touch.

Sarah moved to New York and I moved to Virginia and in the days before cell phones, Twitter and Facebook you could easily lose touch with someone via a lost phone number and a canned voice saying "that number is no longer in service. If you need help, hang up and dial your operator." I would have done so to get Sarah back in my world but like me, my operator had no idea where she had gone.

Besides, I was too distracted to find out. Concentrating on becoming the next Katie Couric I had little time to track down lost friends. So my Sister-cousin–my partner in holiday crime– slipped away from my world, along with at least 3 old boyfriends, 7 neighborhood pals and every single person who signed "friends forever" in my junior high yearbook.

Three decades later my film, the Breast Cancer Diaries, aired on Discovery Health and within a few days I got an email on my film's webpage from a familiar cyber-face: my cousin Sarah. She'd seen the film and felt compelled and excited to be back in my life–having just see my world collapse and watch me fight my way back over 9 months of cancer hell condensed into a tight 72 minute documentary.

I almost cried reading the note. As our Irish luck would have it (our mothers are sisters and both have ties to the Old Sod) I had moved within an hour's plane ride of her. Suddenly, magically, we were back.

It's hard to put into words what our present friendship feels like for me. Though I've never had a long lost twin I can only imagine that this is a scratch-the-surface take on it. When I say that Sarah was my special cousin as a child

I'm not gilding the lily–I'm dead serious. And when we lost touch it was one of those things that when people would say "do you have any regrets?" would pop up in my head, right along with dating that tall dark and dreary guy I wasted a year of my life on post college.

So as I write this blog I am happy to tell you that Sarah and I are about to embark on a trip together. It involves an airplane, a fancy hotel, miles of sandy beaches, and two girlfriends laughing it up. We haven't been side by side holding hands and getting into trouble since we stole Nana's pecan tarts from under Auntie Ann's nose just before Christmas dinner back in 1975. But this friendship, pock-marked with my cancer, her failed marriage and our devastatingly long absence from the other's life, is about to enjoy a rebirth like you read about in What To Expect When You're Expecting.

And just like we used to, I'm expecting that the two of us are going to have a blast.

BECAUSE I CAN
Apr 1, 2011 05:37 PM

When I was little I wore a tiger paw bikini that I loved.

In the late 60's terry cloth suits for kids were the rage and mine, white with a paw shape striped like a jungle cat's fur was my ultimate favorite swim wear. In photos of me and my 5 brother and sisters and 11 cousins clustered around our 4 aunts and uncles, 3 sets of parents and our (maternal) grandparents sitting for cocktails on a Maine beach, the suit features prominently in slides my mother either took or had a beach walker take with her leather-bound Nikkormat camera. Mom, in her paisley cover up and grecian style sandals, wore that thing like jewelry. She loved taking family pictures. And I'm just like her.

But taking a photo of myself in a bikini hasn't happened since those days clustered around my grandpa back at Goose Rocks Beach. I was either too modest or too pregnant to even think of putting on a two piece. Then I got breast cancer and along with it, a double mastectomy. Now I have no breasts–and I don't mean small ones, or fake ones, I mean 'no' ones; nada, zilch, zero. I made the difficult decision to do without a fake pair and just live as I am.

Many times my lack of breasts isn't even noticeable, as I try to stay slim, eat well and exercise. And anything that emphasizes nipples and curves kind of highlights the situation and so has been a no-no on my shopping list. So when a friend recently suggested I bring a bikini to my beach getaway with my cousin, I thought she'd lost her mind. The upper part of a bikini is basically a piece of cloth designed to thinly veil the sexuality beneath it. Assuming you have sexuality beneath it.

Which brings me back to me. I've lived as a breast less woman in America for 7 years now and I've graduated slowly from baggy shirts to high collars to solid print scoops to sleeveless v-necks. Now fighting metastatic breast cancer, I am trying things I've never had the guts for in the past because I'm still here and to put it simply, because I can.

I suppose we all decide we simply can't do things—we're either not smart enough, not tall enough, not brave enough, not rich enough. And maybe that's in part true but in reality, we put a lot more restrictions on our movements than anybody else ever could. Once you tell your mind it's out of the question, then even picking up a pencil is now truly out of your reach.

Blah blah blah—what's my point? My point is that today, 40 years from the last time I did this, I put a bikini on. I borrowed it from that friend who told me I could do it. She even said I should do it. I've been working out and doing my anti-cancer diet and the good news about eating nuts and twigs for a living is that the body doesn't hold onto much fat. And she's right, I'm looking okay these days.

I took the suit, packed it in my bag, and pulled it out and looked at it. But until I told myself I could do it, I still couldn't.

So today, I told myself I could. (see below)

And I hope whatever it is that you've been thinking you can't do, some one of these days you can tell yourself that you can, too.

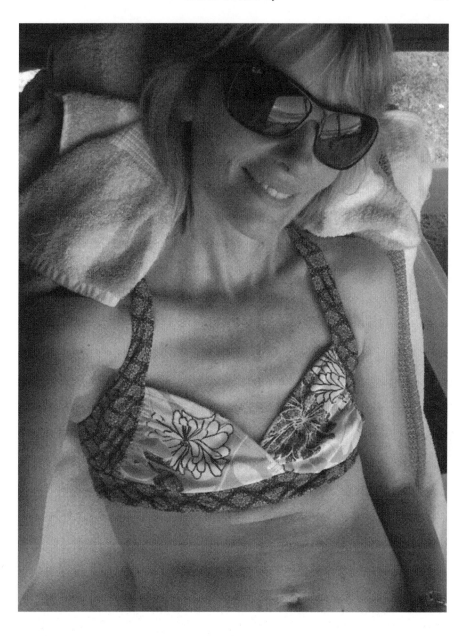

THE FINISH LINE
April 12, 2011 09:47 AM

I was asked the other day how my brother in law Stephen did on his big bike ride that I blogged about in February titled "Motivate"-- the bike ride where you ride all day and night, for 24 hours straight, with a few naps in between to keep your body from exploding from the inside out.

The weather that day for his ride was cold and rainy. I got a text from him at about 5 a.m. his time– 18 hours into the event, saying he'd done what he could and he was ending his quest, about 6 hours short of the 24 hour ending.

I was so proud of him. I still can't even believe he did as much as he did, that he rode that far. He banked about 200 miles peddling his cycle with my photo taped to the front of it, splattered with mud, rain and bugs. I even can't fathom that ride–and technically I was on it.
Sure he didn't actually get to the official 24 hour finish line, but what's a finish line? There's the one the organization sets up for the masses, so everybody knows what's at stake and where they're supposed to go and all that. And then there's the one inside you that tells you what you're able to accomplish, how long you can handle it, and ultimately when you're done, when you need to call it a day. That's *your* finish line, wherever it happens.

And it's the one that matters most, I think, because it's yours. Even though it's socially acceptable to be the one to cross the goal line and get the coveted blue ribbon, only one person gets that. Everybody else gets something else– and it shouldn't be the feeling or the fact that they lost. It should be the knowledge that they did it in the first place– they participated, did their damnedest, tried their hardest. And in my opinion they *did* win –because they showed up in the first place.

As you can imagine, Stephen was tired from the whole race-til-you-can't-race-any-more thing and took a few days to recover. Then he went on to his next thing–which was going down a river in the Grand Canyon on a raft. Like I told you, this guys is an adventure maniac.

Which brings me back to me, only because my first blog compared his quest–to do the 24 hour bike ride–with mine, to make it through my own race for life. Fighting metastatic breast cancer means I don't know how long my race will last, which at its best is depressing and at its worst can paralyze me with fear. But I challenge myself every day to get out and smile, exercise, eat right, laugh, hug, write and embrace every day, because why? Because I can. Like Stephen and his outdoor adventures, we do because we can. And here I am doing it right now, smiling, writing, about to go to a film screening of my film, *The Breast Cancer Diaries*--so today seems to be in the bag.

If I believe what I read in health magazines then my literal finish line should be somewhere around 75 years of age. Yet because I'm fighting metastatic breast cancer and I haven't yet reached 50, I am not sure that's going to happen. Can I make it to 50? How about 55? Do I hear 60?

Like I said, finish lines, while socially created to give us a goal, are really in their most sincerest forms completely personal. It's how far you make it–doing your best, assessing your odds, dealing with bad weather and giving it all you've got that's the real accomplishment. That's what Stephen did during his monster bike ride and I was proud of him for it.

And whenever mine happens, I plan to be proud of myself for getting to my finish line, too.

ABOUT THE AUTHOR

Ann Murray Paige is an award-winning journalist, writer, filmmaker and speaker. Her blog, 'Ann's Diary' at ProjectPinkDiary was named a Top Cancer Blog in 2010. Her film, *The Breast Cancer Diaries*, was honored by the Maine Cancer Foundation and the International Union Against Cancer and has been seen around the world including India, Israel, Canada, Sweden and all of Latin America and has been dubbed into Spanish. She is an expert blogger at Discovery Health and her book, '*pink tips. breast cancer advice from someone who's been there*' earned literary and medical acclaim--being called a book that's 'not just good for breast cancer patients but for anybody going through something tough in life.' She co-founded the non-profit Project Pink with former ABC/CNN correspondent Linda Pattillo and together the two work to spread awareness of young women and breast cancer. Paige sits on the advisory board of the Davis Feminist Film Festival and lives in the San Francisco Bay Area with her husband and two children. Visit Ann at www.annmurraypaige.com